DOC'S FIRST AID GUIDE

Kathleen A. Handal, M.D.

ER Doc

We recently purchased these manuals <u>in French, English, and Spanish</u> as a quick, first aid guide for our company's international project sites. We operate in well over 40 countries and Dr. Handal's "Doc's First Aid Guide," is an easy-to-read, compact, and comprehensive guide to a myriad of ailments and health issues that may arise no matter where you may be located. We feel that this manual will better equip our personnel to deal with daily first aid issues that may come to pass and we highly recommend this guide to others.
Becca, Abt Associates

"Invaluable e-book ... valuable resources that make a contribution to improving family health and safety ... concise guide takes out all of the guess work, telling the reader exactly what to do and what not to do when first aid situations arise."
Sari Fine Shepphird, Ph.D. Psychologist & Author

"Key is on the cover - Read it before you need it ... Helps decide what you can do at home and when you need to seek more advanced help."
Claire Merrick

"Very valuable and accessible contribution to the education needed for first aid responses."
Delores Rogers

"Replaces that old, heavy reference book."
Stephanie Herold

Published by DocHandal, LLC

Copyright © 2009, by Kathleen A. Handal, M.D.
Updated 1/2018

ISBN-13: 978-0-9827131-9-8

DocHandal, LLC publishes first aid, health and safety materials in a variety of formats. Discounts for bulk orders and customized editions may be available from the publisher.

Visit http://www.DocHandal.com for more information.

Printed in the USA

DISCLAIMER: This is a guide until medical assistance is obtained. The author does not represent that every acceptable first aid/medical procedure is contained herein or those abnormal or unusual circumstances may not warrant or require additional procedures. This material is not designed to take the place of first aid training by qualified instructors or evaluation by a physician. DocHandal recommends formal first aid & CPR training for everyone.

The information within this guide is a compilation of general medical first aid, reflecting the current knowledge and accepted emergency practice in the United States at the time this guide was published. The reader is urged to stay informed of changes in emergency care procedures.

ABOUT THE AUTHOR

Kathleen Handal, MD is a nationally and internationally known emergency medicine "Doc". She authored *"The American Red Cross First Aid & Safety Handbook"*, which was written for the lay audience.

Doc believes physicians have a responsibility to teach and share medical common sense. Her website, *www.dochandal.com*, serves as a base for her many consumer education endeavors. A frequent host and co-host on talk-radio health shows, she has also appeared on CNN and the Today Show. Her *"Medical Emergencies in the Workplace"* video won a bronze medal in the International Cindy Competition and was a Telly Award finalist. She has co-authored a series of medical textbooks.

As part of her dedication to public education, Doc wrote, directed and produced *"Trauma Run"*, a nationally distributed video for grades 2-6. The video, produced in Spanish and English, teaches children how to respond to a medical emergency when no adults are available.

Doc's First Aid Guide is available in French and Spanish versions. In *"Your ER Guide"*, Doc provides valuable insight into how an emergency room operates, so you'll know how to get the best care possible. It's like having Doc Handal at your side when you need her the most.

Acknowledgments

Many thanks to Brian Coonce, Barbara O'Neill-Maguire, BSN, RN, OCN, Anita Kaul, Barbi Neary, RRT and all my ER patients over the years for their many and varied contributions, not the least of which was patience and trust.

CONTENTS

MAKING A DIFFERENCE

The steps a rescuer takes during the first few minutes of a medical emergency are critical - they can mean the difference between temporary or permanent disability or between life and death. That's why first aid knowledge and training are so important. They prepare you to intervene calmly and effectively in a medical emergency. Everyone has a chance to be a life saver.

In this book you'll find easy-to-follow instructions on how to help in the more common medical emergencies. You'll learn what to do and what not to do if you're the first one on the scene. So, familiarize yourself with this material before an incident occurs. And keep in mind that reading this information is no substitute for formal instruction and practice. Not every possible medical emergency situation is presented in this guide.

Before you become a rescuer, be aware of your own sensitivities and physical limitations. If you are not cut out for hands-on help at the scene of a medical emergency, you can still aid. The fact that you know how to get help and can communicate effectively will make a difference.

It's also important to exercise compassion and understanding for the victim's situation. Your job is to stay calm and to reassure the victim without making false promises. Always remember to give the victim as much privacy as possible, including asking observers to act as a screen by facing out from the situation. Again, thinking ahead about these details and the role you might play will make a difference in ensuring the effectiveness of your assistance.

READ THIS BOOK BEFORE YOU NEED IT!

In this book you will see how to:

- Size up the situation
- Set priorities
- Perform cardiopulmonary resuscitation (CPR) and use the Automated External Defibrillator (AED)
- Administer first aid for specific emergencies
- Create an Emergency Info Sheet
- Put together a First Aid Kit, using Doc Handal's First Aid Kit Checklist

NOTE: Any word in *bold italic* in this book can be referenced from the Table of Contents.

First aid is serious.
Dedicate some time to learning how to help. Any time you spend doing this is time well spent. Make sure you have a first aid kit at home, in your car and at work. Familiarize yourself with its contents. Replace and update supplies as needed. You want to be ready to act quickly and correctly in a medical emergency.

1. SIZE UP THE SITUATION

Your first step in a medical emergency, before attempting a rescue, must be to look around and ask yourself "Is the scene safe for me?". Too often well-intentioned rescuers become victims themselves when they risk their own safety to help others. Don't think that rushing in will make you a hero. If the area is unsafe, go for help or put on the personal protective equipment (PPE) that will permit you to assist safely.

Keep in mind that blood and body fluids may contain infectious matter, so ALWAYS take **Universal Precautions,** like wearing gloves or a CPR barrier mask, to protect yourself. Barrier devices should be kept in your **First Aid Kit.**

2. SET PRIORITIES

After you've determined that it is safe for you to enter the area, approach the victim. As you do, look for signs of life. Tap the victim on the shoulder and ask, "Are you OK?" (Saying "OK" is internationally understood.) Determine if the victim is breathing.

If a spine or neck injury is suspected, don't move the victim unless there's a threat of fire, explosion or other life-threatening danger. If a victim is face down, turn the victim face up. If a spine injury is suspected, use the Log-Roll Technique to turn the victim.

- **If the victim does not respond, CALL FOR MEDICAL HELP, and, if not breathing, send someone to get an AED and start CPR.**
- **If the victim responds, identify yourself as willing to assist. Find out what is wrong and take steps to help the victim. Always treat the more serious injuries first. It's important to stay calm and assure the victim while you're performing first aid measures.**

CALLING FOR MEDICAL HELP

How you call for help should be another consideration. In most cases, the victim will need some type of emergency medical help, be it from Emergency Medical Technicians (EMTs), the company nurse or a physician at the hospital. If you're not alone, tell someone else to go for medical assistance while you help the victim. In an emergency, it's important to remember that every minute counts.

When alone, in certain circumstances, intervention is your priority. However, it is usually best to call Emergency Medical Services (EMS) before you intervene, especially if you witness a collapse or come across an unresponsive victim.

The number varies worldwide: 911 in the USA/Canada, 999 in many other countries, including the United Kingdom, Hong Kong, and Singapore. In Australia 000 or 112 from all GSM mobile phones or 106 to the text-based relay service. Not all areas in USA support 911 texting. Check for changes in your area.

When you call EMS, remember that there are certain things a dispatcher will need to know in order to get help to you quickly:

- The address and location of the emergency (including cross streets and specific directions to the exact location of the emergency).

- Your name, phone number and the number of a nearby phone.

- A description of what happened and how many people need help. (It's also a good idea to check the victim for medical information jewelry and to report findings to the dispatcher.)

Stay on the phone until the dispatcher tells you it's okay to hang up. Remain calm and listen carefully—the dispatcher may give you valuable first aid instructions, including how to perform CPR.

When seconds count, an **Emergency Info Sheet (EIS)** is a great timesaver. Take the time now to fill in the emergency numbers. Make a copy of this call sheet and post it next to the telephones in your work area and at home. Having this information handy will help you obtain emergency medical assistance quickly.

In addition, make sure your cell phone directory includes the entry "ICE" (In Case of Emergency). ICE is the person you want to be called if you're ill or injured. Emergency personnel are trained to look for this number when they need to gather information about a victim.

UNIVERSAL PRECAUTIONS

Anyone involved in the care of an ill or injured person can be at risk for acquiring an infectious disease, such as hepatitis, tuberculosis, acquired immune deficiency syndrome (AIDS) or meningitis. Identifying a person as having a communicable disease can be difficult or impossible; therefore, rescuers must presume everyone is a risk. Always take protective measures to avoid coming in contact with another person's body fluids (blood, urine, sputum or secretions). Protective measures should also be taken during cleanup and disposal of materials used to care for the victim.

To reduce the risk of infection, follow these guidelines:
- Always cover all open skin areas.

- Wear the appropriate personal protective equipment (PPE), such as gloves, masks, CPR barrier masks (when giving rescue breathing) and goggles.
- If possible, place a barrier between you and the victim's body fluids.
- Minimize the splashing of body fluids.
- Wash hands (even if you were wearing gloves) and any exposed area with soap and water immediately after providing care.
- Handle sharp objects with caution.
- Wear a mask if there's a risk of exposure to airborne disease.
- Dispose of contaminated PPE in an appropriate container.

Contact your *Primary Care Physician* (PCP) immediately if you come in direct contact with another's body fluids, especially if you have concerns.

3. CPR

If a person is unresponsive (appears lifeless, doesn't move, and doesn't respond to your shout or a tap on the shoulder) and not breathing, you need to start CPR right away. Gasping is not breathing! Yell for someone to call EMS and get an AED. An AED applied quickly may restart the heart. Don't worry, AEDs are user friendly and I've included instructions on how to operate one.

- Understand that when a victim's heart has stopped pumping blood (cardiac arrest), permanent brain damage can occur in six minutes, so you must act fast.

- Cardiac arrest can strike at any age and may be caused by many conditions, including heart attack, suffocation, allergic reaction, drowning, choking or electric shock.

What a rescuer should do when CPR is needed depends on training. If you are not trained in CPR, you should start chest compressions immediately and follow instructions given by an EMS dispatcher. If you are CPR trained and able, you should begin with chest compressions and then add rescue breathing, following current CPR guidelines. Research has shown that when chest compressions are given immediately to a cardiac arrest (unresponsive/not breathing) victim, the chance of survival is improved.

I'm going to explain how to perform **Chest-Compression-Only CPR** on an adult for those who have never taken a CPR or Heartsaver® class. And then, since I always recommend formal training in CPR, I'm going to review the basics of what is covered in a CPR class for those who have taken one.

If you've never taken a CPR class, you should still read the **CPR Basics** section. Being familiar with this information will be helpful in case an EMS dispatcher ever has to guide you through these lifesaving techniques.

NOTE: Healthcare providers, such as nurses and paramedics, learn more detailed instructions than what is covered in this book.

CHEST-COMPRESSION-ONLY CPR

- Be sure you are safe.

- Tap and shout "Are you OK?" to assess responsiveness, and look to see if the victim is breathing - gasping is NOT breathing.

- If unresponsive, have someone call EMS and get an AED while you start chest compressions.

- Position the victim flat on a firm surface with the head at the same level as the heart. Open chest clothing.

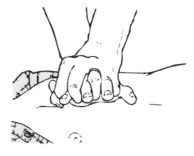

- Kneel facing the victim's chest. Place the heel of your hand on the center of chest – the lower half of breastbone/sternum.

- Place the heel of your other hand on top of the hand on the chest. With shoulders back, straighten your arms, lean directly over the person and lock your elbows.

- Use straight-down pressure through both arms, push the breastbone down toward the spine, at least 2 in./5 cm. Push hard and fast at a rate of 100 - 120 compressions per minute (100 -120/min.). Allow chest to recoil between compressions. This is hard work. Don't lean between compressions and don't stop compressions unless necessary.

- You may be directed by an EMS dispatcher to perform rescue breaths.

o   If a CPR barrier mask isn't available and you have any worries about giving rescue breathing or consider the victim at high risk for disease transmission, say so. Your own safety is a priority.

NOTE: CPR on infants and children has better outcomes when chest compressions are combined with rescue breathing. This is best learned in a CPR class.

CPR CLASS BASICS

Remember, proper functioning of the heart and lungs is basic to life. Monitoring responsiveness, which includes determining whether the person is breathing and their heart is pumping, takes priority over other illnesses and injuries. Because, let's face it: if you're not breathing and your heart isn't beating, having a stabilized fractured bone isn't going to make much difference.

A trained lay rescuer (someone who has taken a CPR class) should provide, at a minimum, chest compressions. Rescue breaths can be added at a ratio of 30 compressions to 2 breaths. So, if you find someone who is unresponsive, start right in with chest compressions and provide rescue breaths as you've been trained.

It's correct to think Compression, Airway and Breathing (C-A-B) instead of Airway, Breathing and Circulation (A-B-C) when it comes to an unresponsive victim. However, if you're monitoring someone who is having a seizure, for example, monitoring the person's breathing is most important. Use your common sense and prioritize when it comes to monitoring a victim.

Remember, CPR involves the use of chest compressions and rescue breathing. During CPR, the trained rescuer attempts to maintain a steady flow of oxygen and blood for the victim, whose lungs and heart have stopped functioning. It is best administered by a trained person. Remember:

        C - Chest Compressions
        A - Airway
        B - Breathing

Here are the basics of single rescuer CPR for an adult:

•   Do not move the victim if you suspect a back or neck injury, unless to restore breathing or circulation—and then only use the *Log-Roll Technique* so the person moves as a unit.

- Do not tilt the head back to open the airway of a victim with a possible neck or spine injury.

- Do not press on the soft tissue of chin or neck during *Rescue Breathing*.

C - COMPRESSIONS

To perform chest compressions on an adult:

- Position the victim flat on a firm surface with the head at the same level as the heart. Open chest clothing.

- Kneel facing the victim's chest. Place the heel of your hand on the center of chest – the lower half of breastbone/sternum. Then, place your other hand on top. With shoulders back, straighten your arms, lean directly over the person and lock your elbows.

- Use straight-down pressure through both arms to push breastbone down toward the spine, at least 2 in./5 cm. Push hard and fast at rate of 100-120 compressions per minute.

- Release pressure after each compression, but don't let your hands come off the victim's chest. Do not pause between compressions. The compressions should be smooth, regular and uninterrupted. Compression and relaxation time should be equal.

- After 30 compressions, breathe twice into the victim's mouth (each breath lasting 1 second).

FYI: Healthcare professionals are trained to check for a pulse. I think it is important for you to understand how this is done.

PULSE CHECK

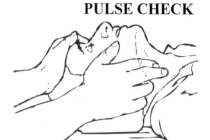

- Using your fingers (not thumb), gently feel the carotid artery on the victim's neck for at least 5 seconds and no more than 10 seconds to find a pulse. (To find the carotid artery, put two fingers on the victim's Adam's apple [larynx]. Slide your fingers to the side and direct them into the groove between the windpipe and the muscle at the side of the neck. This is where the carotid artery is located.) Gently feel for a pulse.

IF PULSE IS PRESENT BUT THERE IS NO BREATHING - Perform ***Rescue Breathing*** at a rate of one breath every 5-6 seconds (10-12/min) until breathing is restored or help arrives. Suspect opioid use when this occurs; an antidote, naloxone, is available as an auto-injector and in a nasal spray.

REMEMBER: IF NO PULSE IS PRESENT - and medical help has been called, continue Chest Compressions until *AED* arrives, help arrives or the victim moves.

A - AIRWAY

Sometimes an obstruction has caused the victim to stop breathing. This is how to open an airway and clear an obstruction to prepare for rescue breathing:

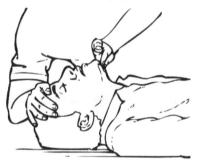

- The most common cause of airway obstruction is the tongue. To keep the airway open, perform the "head-tilt, chin-lift". Place one hand on the victim's forehead and put the fingers of your other hand under the bony part of the chin. Press down on the forehead and lift the chin out so that the mouth is slightly open. If you suspect a spinal injury, do not press down on the forehead nor tilt the head back, simply perform a chin lift. The victim may start to breathe after you open the airway. If the victim is breathing and no spine injury is suspected, place the victim in the ***Recovery Position***.

- If an obstruction to the airway is **visible and reachable** and the victim is unconscious, remove the object with your fingers. (Gloves should be worn.)

- Never place your fingers in the mouth of a conscious or semiconscious individual. If the victim is conscious, give first aid for *Choking*.

B - BREATHING

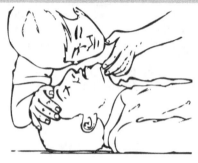

If the airway is clear, check breathing. Place your ear above the victim's mouth and nose. Watch for signs of breathing. Gasping is not breathing. If the victim isn't breathing, start *Rescue Breathing*. (Use a barrier device if one is available.) If you have any reservations about giving rescue breathing or consider the victim to be at high risk for disease transmission, perform *Chest-Compression-Only CPR*.

RESCUE BREATHING

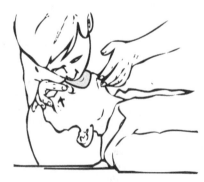

- Pinch the victim's nose to close nostrils, keeping the airway open by the head-tilt, chin-lift.

- Take a deep breath and seal your lips around the outside of the victim's mouth, preferably with a CPR barrier mask, creating an airtight seal.

- Give the victim 2 full breaths (1 second each), taking your lips off the victim's mouth to inhale between each breath.

- Check for chest rising and falling with each breath you give. The rising of the chest during your exhalations indicates the effectiveness of your breaths.

- Perform 5 sets of the 30 compressions and 2 breaths within 2 minutes.

- Continue CPR until an *AED* is applied, the person starts to move, help arrives or until you can no longer continue.

AUTOMATED EXTERNAL DEFIBRILLATOR (AED)

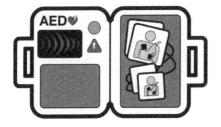

CPR alone is not always enough to restart the heart. AEDs save lives if used right away for certain types of cardiac arrests. This computerized medical device analyzes the heart and delivers electric shock (defibrillation) when needed through connected adhesive pads. The AED and you work through visual and audio prompts. Instructions are simple and directions are given one step at a time.

The EMS dispatcher may tell you where the nearest AED is located and instruct you to send for it. AEDs are common in public places and also carried to the scene by trained responders. Smartphone Apps for some locales show the nearest AED and trained citizens willing to respond. Survival of victims is based on the time it takes to start CPR and defibrillation. Therefore, until the AED arrives, chest compressions should be done by pushing fast and hard on the chest. When an AED is available, lay rescuers should perform CPR while it is being applied.

Good to Know:
- Defibrillation can only save a heart stopped by specific rhythms.
- Pads for children 1 to 8 years of age are clearly marked.
- If the victim has lots of hair on his chest, remove the hair by applying an adhesive pad. Press down firmly and remove the pad with hair attached. Apply a fresh adhesive pad to hairless area.
- Chest muscles may jerk when a shock is delivered.

What an AED does:
- Recognizes cardiac arrest from rhythms that requires electrical shock
- Warns when a shock is needed
- Gives a shock if needed
- Tells you to "stand clear" from the victim for your safety

- Do not use an AED if victim is lying in water.
- Do not use an AED if chest is covered with sweat or water.
- Do not put an AED pad over a medication patch, remove patch with glove and wipe area before applying AED pad.
- Do not place an AED pad over a pacemaker (hard lump under chest skin).
- Do not touch a victim when AED says to ""stand clear"" or while delivering a shock.
- Do not use an AED on infants less than 12 months of age.
- Do not use adult pads on children under age 8.

- If unresponsive and not breathing, apply AED quickly. Visual displays show where to place the two adhesive pads on the victim's chest. Follow the voice prompts. You'll be instructed to "stand clear" while the machine is analyzing whether or not a shock is necessary.
- If delivery of a shock is required, you'll be prompted to "stand clear" again. If other people are on the scene, make sure no one is touching the victim. The machine will tell you when it is delivering a shock. Some devices instruct you to press the button to deliver the shock.
- The AED may also instruct you to start CPR.
- Perform CPR for 2 minutes and reapply the AED.

4. FIRST AID

Making a decision about calling for emergency medical help is usually one of the first things you do when you come upon the scene of a medical emergency. Obviously, some minor injuries may not require calling EMS or even a visit to a medical facility. Treatment can be given on the scene, and no further medical attention will be required unless complications arise. Here are some more tips to remember about providing first aid:

- A victim can often be safely transported to the hospital by a co-worker or friend. However, whenever you're unsure of what to do, or feel that emergency assistance is needed, don't hesitate to call EMS.

- Giving first aid should never delay activating EMS or getting medical attention when required.

- Attention to monitoring the victim and performing CPR to the level you are trained is always important while administering first aid.

- A well-stocked first aid kit is often the key to providing the right help. Make sure your kits contain the items listed in the *First Aid Kit Checklist.*

Remember, Do No Further Harm - If you are unsure or your intervention causes pain at any time, stop.

- Check to make sure the scene is safe before you approach.
- Introduce yourself and ask for permission to help.
- Determine what the problem is and what type of help is needed.
- Call EMS if someone is seriously ill, injured or you are unsure of what to do.

For each first aid situation listed, there is a description of the problem, a list of signs and symptoms and instruction on what to do and not do in each situation. What to do may require a *First Aid Kit*, so be sure to take it with you.

ALLERGIC REACTION

Many agents - including foods, venom, drugs, chemicals and other substances - can cause reactions that range from mild to severe and life-threatening. The progressive reaction can appear within minutes of exposure or may show up hours later. The more serious reactions usually develop within minutes of the victim's exposure to the allergen. Many who know they have severe allergies carry a prescribed epinephrine auto-injector (usually with 2 doses) to counter the reaction.

SIGNS & SYMPTOMS:
Mild Reaction
- Itching, raised, red skin, rash and hives
- Itching around eyes
- Swelling at a bite/sting mark
- Stuffy nose, sneezing

Severe Reaction
- Swelling of the throat, face and eyes
- Difficulty breathing
- Fainting and *Shock*
- Loss of consciousness

- Do not pick up animals that can bite or sting.
- Do not rub or squeeze irritated area.
- Do not apply a tourniquet.
- Do not squeeze out a stinger.
- Do not harass or tease any animals.
- Do not elevate body part that has been bitten or stung.
- Do not stop person from taking own medication for allergic reaction.
- Do not give the victim anything by mouth other than their allergy medication.
- Do not make a victim vomit after eating food that he or she is allergic to.

- If reaction is severe, get medical help immediately.
- Identify the allergen.
- Help the victim administer their own medication for allergic reaction.
- Monitor for responsiveness and breathing.
- Monitor and treat for *Shock* if present.

Epinephrine Auto-injector

Here's how to use:
- Take off the safety cap; do not touch either end.
- Hold in fist at 90° angle to victim's outer mid-thigh, not the buttock.
- Jab the tip firmly against thigh (OK to inject through clothing).
- Hold firmly in place for 10 seconds; a small amount of medication may remain.
- Remove and rub the spot for 10 seconds. Note time.
- If not resolved and no medical help is likely in 5-10 minutes, a second dose may be considered
- Stay with victim until medical help arrives.
- Dispose of auto-injector properly.

Allergic Reactions also under *Bites/Stings.*

AMPUTATION

When a body part is partially or completely amputated, quick action is required to help ensure the best possible repair. Tissue can be preserved for up to 18 hours if properly cared for. Reattachment can be done up to 24 hours after amputation; however, successful reattachment has the best chance of occurring within 4 to 6 hours of amputation.

- Do not make the judgment that the body part is too small or too damaged to be reattached.
- Do not throw away any body part, no matter how small.
- Do not separate amputated part from victim.
- Do not place amputated part directly on ice or in water.
- Do not use dry ice to preserve a severed body part.

- Check for responsiveness and breathing.
- Give first aid for *Bleeding.*
- Monitor and treat for *Shock*, if present.
- Care for Amputated Part(s)
    - Clean amputated part, if necessary, with sterile or clean water, then cover and wrap in sterile dressing.
    - Place in a plastic bag and seal.
    - Place bag in another container with ice or ice plus water. Label with victim's name.
- Keep the amputated part with the victim at all times.

BITES / STINGS

Insect, snake and spider bites and stings are usually minor but can result in illness and disease transmission, for example, Lyme disease, Zika and West Nile virus. Certain snake, scorpion, and spider stings/bites can introduce life-threatening venom into our bodies. Usually what caused a bite or sting is unknown, so let the signs and symptoms direct you to getting proper care; it is not necessary to know the cause. Animal and human bites that break the skin introduce germs, so first aid care is important. Rabies from bats and wild animal bites is also a consideration.

Lyme disease is spread by ticks, which are extremely tiny. Most victims aren't aware they have been bitten. Only a blood test can determine if you have Lyme disease. If the results are positive, treatment with antibiotics is required. When Lyme disease is left untreated, the victim runs the risk of being stricken with crippling arthritis and neurological and heart irregularities.

Get Medical Help For:
- Tick bites
- Rashes, typically a bulls-eye pattern
- Fever
- Stiff joints
- Chronic fatigue
- Flu-like symptoms

West Nile virus and **Zika virus** are transmitted by infected mosquitoes. Only a blood test can determine if you are ill from the West Nile or Zika virus. There is no medicine at this time, but a human vaccine may be available in the future.

Get Medical Help For:
- Headache with neck stiffness
- High fever, rash
- Tremors, muscle weakness
- Convulsion/seizure
- Vision loss
- Numbness, paralysis

Prevention is the best medicine! Know what hazards are common in your area and how to avoid them!

- Do not elevate body part that has been bitten or stung.
- Do not stop person from taking their own medication.
- Do not rub or squeeze an irritated area.
- Do not apply a tourniquet.
- Do not use suction to remove venom.
- Do not try to squeeze out a stinger.

- Do not remove a tick using your hand, rubbing alcohol, a match, gasoline or nail polish.
- Do not try to catch what bit you; time spent doing so delays treatment.

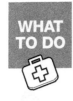

- Monitor for responsiveness.
- Help the victim administer medication for allergic reaction. Assist with *Epinephrine Auto-injector*, as needed.
- Apply cold compresses to wound to relieve pain and swelling.
- Watch for signs of severe *Allergic Reaction.*
- Control *Bleeding* if needed.
- If the sting was inflicted by a honeybee and the stinger is still in the skin, remove it by scraping with a plastic card, knife, or razor blade. Don't squeeze the stinger, or the venom sac will send a new supply of venom into the bloodstream.
- If a tick is embedded in the skin, it must be killed before it is removed in one piece. Get medical help for proper removal.
- If an animal is involved, and it's believed to be venomous, try to photograph it. Call **Poison Help Center at 1-800-222-1222,** accessible 24/7 in the USA.
- Watch for signs of wound infection.
- Get medical help if needed.

For animal or human bites that break the skin:
- Make sure the scene is safe. (Avoid animals acting strangely, including humans.)
- Wearing gloves, clean the wound with soap and lots of running water.
- Then stop *Bleeding* by applying pressure.
- Report all animal bites to the police/animal control.
- If there's bruising or swelling, place a cold pack (mixture ice/water) wrapped in cloth on area for up to 20 minutes, or until medical help is obtained.
- Get medical help for infection prevention.
- A tetanus booster may be required.

BLEEDING

External bleeding you can see, while internal bleeding you cannot. Both will require medical attention. The seriousness of an external wound doesn't always correspond to the size of the wound or the amount of blood lost. For example, a small superficial scalp wound may bleed heavily because of the rich blood supply to the head. Bleeding from an artery is more serious and will take longer to stop. You may only see signs on the outside of the body, such as bruising and swelling, indicating a bleeding injury inside the body. Here's more information about bleeding that you need to know:

- You have approximately 5.7 liters of blood in your body. This amount is needed to maintain circulation. Rapidly losing just one liter can result in **Shock** or death. That's why a victim's pulse will quicken and then weaken as blood is lost. If someone is bleeding heavily, it's important for you to stay calm, control the bleeding and get medical help immediately.

- Internal bleeding is hard to detect. There may not be any pain. Suspect it if someone has experienced trauma, even a slight trauma for someone on blood thinning medications. Weakness, paleness and a faint pulse are all signs of internal bleeding. Prompt medical attention is needed.

- Small scrapes or surface cuts that have stopped bleeding heal better when cleaned, protected with antibiotic cream and kept covered.

- As a result of injury, medication and certain medical conditions can cause organs to bleed internally, causing pain, loss of consciousness and even death.

EXTERNAL BLEEDING

SIGNS & SYMPTOMS:
- Blood flowing out of body
- Spurts of blood indicate an artery is torn

- Do not apply a tourniquet *unless trained* to do so.
- Do not push anything back into the skin.
- Do not apply antibiotic cream unless wound is minor and cleaned first.
- Do not remove blood-soaked bandage.
- Do not put pressure on an object sticking out of a wound.
- Do not use pressure points or elevation.
- Do not allow blood-saturated dressing over chest wound to become an occlusive dressing.

Wounds - Major Bleeding

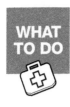

- Call for medical help.
- Apply continuous firm, direct pressure to wound, using clean cloth or bandage for 5 minutes without lifting to see if stopped.
- If bleeding soaks through bandage:
    - o Do not remove the original bandage.
    - o Apply more bandages and pressure or tourniquet if trained.
- Get medical help to cleanse and close the wound.
- Monitor and treat for *Shock*, if present.

Wounds - Minimal Bleeding

- Clean the wound with soap and copious amounts of clean running tap water until foreign matter is removed.
- Apply continuous firm, direct pressure to wound until bleeding stops.
- Once the bleeding stops, apply antibiotic ointment. Cover with dressing.
- If bleeding soaks through bandage:
    - o Do not remove the original bandage.
    - o Apply more bandages and pressure.

For Impaled Objects - Object Stuck In Body Part

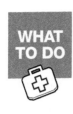

- Call for medical help.
- Stabilize the impaled object to prevent any movement. Even a small amount of movement can cause serious internal damage. If required, stabilize with multiple dressings until secure.
- To control bleeding, apply direct pressure around the wound.
- Monitor and treat for *Shock*, if present.

See *Impaled Object in Eye*

INTERNAL BLEEDING

SIGNS & SYMPTOMS:
- Nausea
- Cold, clammy skin
- Trouble breathing after an injury
- Abdominal pain, tenderness

- Spitting or coughing blood
- Bloody vomit or diarrhea (also may appear like coffee grounds)
- Loss of consciousness with no visible cause
- Signs of *Shock*

BE SUSPECT if any of the above signs and symptoms accompanies:
- An injury to chest or abdomen
- A shooting or stabbing wound
- Car accident, fall from height or pedestrian injury
- Sports injury

- Do not give anything by mouth.
- Do not leave victim alone unless going for help.

- Be sure the scene is safe for you to enter.
- Call for medical help.
- If not nauseated/vomiting and spinal injury is not suspected – place victim in *Shock Position.*
- If nauseated/vomiting and spinal injury is not suspected – place victim in *Recovery Position*.
- Monitor and treat for *Shock*, if present.
- Monitor for responsiveness and perform *CPR*, if needed.

BONE / JOINT / MUSCLE INJURIES

Bone, joint and muscle injuries are common, especially among athletes and the elderly. It can be difficult to determine if an injury is a fracture, sprain or strain, so treat all injuries as severe until proven otherwise. Here's some more information that should help you identify the injury and administer the first aid:

- A rupture is a complete tearing of a ligament, tendon or muscle.
- Bruises are swelling, pain and bleeding below the skin, resulting from a direct blow to the area. Discoloration from bleeding under skin can last for days and change colors with time.
- Hematomas arise when large amounts of blood collect under the skin because of tissue injury damage.
- With **Open Fractures**, the broken bone comes through the skin.
- With **Closed Fractures**, the skin over the broken bone remains intact. An x-ray is needed to determine if a fracture has occurred.
- **Sprains and Strains** are ligament and tendon injuries that occur more often than fractures.

- **Sprains** occur at joints from a twisting injury which causes ligament(s) to partially or completely tear or overstretch. An x-ray may be needed to determine if a fracture or sprain exists. Treat as a Fracture until confirmed.
- **Strains** are a tearing or overstretching of a muscle. They typically occur near where the muscle tapers into a tendon and connects to a bone.

FRACTURES

SIGNS & SYMPTOMS:
- Almost immediate swelling and bruising of a bone area
- Inability to normally move affected area
- Pain and tenderness over bone
- Deformity
- Exposed bone ends

- Do not force anyone to use a painful body part.
- Do not straighten a misshapen bone.
- Do not place ice/cold pack directly on skin.
- Do not move victim if neck or spine injury is suspected, unless absolutely necessary.
- Do not move until injury has been immobilized.
- Do not remove shoes, boots or clothes around a possible fracture.
- Splinting is unnecessary if victim can give the broken bone sufficient support and immobility.
- Do not splint a possible fractured bone if doing so causes pain.

SPLINTING

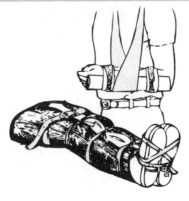

You can learn different splinting techniques in a first aid course. Below are some of the basics of splinting you can use if help is not on the way and moving is necessary.

WHAT TO DO

- Support both sides of the fracture when you lift the fractured limb into the splint. If, for example, you use a newspaper to splint a fractured forearm, be sure to extend the newspaper from the hand to the elbow so that it includes the joint above and below the fracture site.
- Always check circulation of the injured extremity before and after splinting. Note the color of the skin beforehand.
- A splint is probably too tight if the color of the skin changes. Loosen the splint ties until the color improves. If the victim complains of numbness or if swelling occurs, loosen the splint.
- Get medical attention immediately.

CLOSED FRACTURE

(Broken bone doesn't break skin)

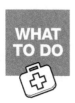

WHAT TO DO

- Call for medical help if the bone is abnormally bent.
- Stabilize the injured area in position found. Splint if necessary.
- Apply cold pack (mixture ice/water) through a barrier directly to area for up to 20 minutes at a time or until uncomfortable.
- Elevate the injured area if it can be immobilized and does not cause more pain.
- Get medical attention.

OPEN FRACTURE

(Broken bone breaks skin)

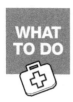

WHAT TO DO

- Call for medical help.
- If necessary, control ***Bleeding*** by applying continuous pressure above the fracture site.
- Cover open wound with dry sterile dressing.
- Stabilize the injured area in position found. ***Splint*** if necessary.
- Monitor and treat for ***Shock***, if present.

SPRAINS / STRAINS

(Joint Injury / Muscle Injury)

SIGNS & SYMPTOMS:
- Swelling and bruising that develops immediately or with time
- Able to use injured part BUT painful
- Pain, soreness and tenderness

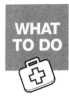

- Seek medical help if unable to bear own weight or if you suspect *Fracture*.
- If necessary, control *Bleeding* by applying continuous firm pressure above the injured site. Cover with sterile dressing.
- Stabilize the injured area in position found. *Splint* if necessary.
- Apply the RICE guidelines: Rest, Ice, Compress and Elevate. Ice is a cold pack (mixture ice/water) placed through a barrier directly to area for up to 20 minutes or until uncomfortable. Reusable gel packs do not cool as well.

BREATHING PROBLEMS

Breathing problems can be caused by a number of conditions, including: heart disease, lung infection (pneumonia), a collapsed lung, asthma, smoking, inhalation of fumes, choking and a chest or head injury. Sudden onset of asthma-like symptoms should be treated with the victim's rescue inhaler. Fear, panic and anxiety may also cause breathing problems, resulting in rapid, shallow breathing, known as hyperventilation or over-breathing. Over-breathing may also occur in more serious medical conditions, including heart attack, bleeding, fever or serious infection.

SIGNS & SYMPTOMS:
- Pale and/or blue face, lips or nail beds
- Noisy breathing, wheezing
- Cough
- Inability to catch breath or shortness of breath
- Very slow or rapid breathing
- Pain while taking a breath

- Do not ignore someone over-breathing.
- Do not force victim into an uncomfortable position.

- Sit the victim upright with support.
- Loosen clothing.
- If on medication for breathing problems, help with medications.
- If a known history of over-breathing from anxiety exists, speak calmly and attempt stress reduction by identifying the fear. Direct victim to a quiet place.
- Reassure and remain with victim until improved.
- If breathing does not return to normal shortly, get medical help.

FUME INHALATION

Injury from inhaling fumes can be sudden or delayed. In a fire, victims are often overcome by smoke inhalation before the flames reach them. In other situations, damage to the lungs may not be evident for 36 hours after exposure. Children and the elderly are most vulnerable. Dangerous fumes arise from car exhaust, cleaning solvents and other everyday chemicals. The type of fume and the duration of exposure will determine the extent of the damage.

SIGNS & SYMPTOMS:
- Burns around mouth or neck
- Soot in nostrils or phlegm
- Singed hairs around nose
- Hoarse voice or no voice at all
- Wheezing
- Drooling or dribbling
- Noisy breathing, gasping for breath
- Burning sensation upon inhaling
- Confusion, disorientation

- Do not make a rescue attempt that puts your own life at risk.
- Never enter a room filled with smoke from a fire.
- Do not go into a fume-filled building without proper gear.

WHAT TO DO

- Call for medical help.
- Remove from source of exposure.
- Monitor for responsiveness and breathing.
- Treat ***Chemical Burns***, if present.
- If victim can sit upright, ask them to take slow, deep breaths.
- Check for other injuries while waiting for help.
- All suspected inhalation injuries require medical attention.

BURNS

Burns can be painful or painless. The severity of a burn may not be obvious for up to 24 hours, and infection may occur if improperly treated. There are three degrees of burns, going from superficial to deep. Sources of burns include heat, chemicals and electricity.

Here's what you need to know:

- Any burn area greater than one percent of the body - approximately the size of the victim's hand - requires medical attention.
- Burns of the fingers, toes, genitals and eyes <u>always</u> require medical attention.
- Burns involving the face, airway and neck are considered life threatening and require immediate medical attention.
- All third-degree burns, no matter how small, require medical attention.
- Anyone who inhales smoke, fumes or flames (***Fume Inhalation***) is also at risk and requires prompt medical attention.
- Remember, heat may cause the airway to swell, resulting in ***Breathing Difficulty***. If you suspect airway burns, get prompt medical attention for the victim while monitoring for responsiveness and breathing.

First-Degree Burns

SIGNS & SYMPTOMS:
- Redness of skin
- Pain
- Mild swelling

WHAT TO DO

- If possible, hold the burned area under cold (not ice cold) running water for at least 10 minutes. Continue until pain subsides.
- Leave uncovered. Protect from sun, dirt and friction.
- Re-examine in 24 hours and look for signs of second-degree burn.
- Medical attention may be required, depending on

location.

Second-Degree Burns

SIGNS & SYMPTOMS:
- Deep reddening of skin
- Blisters
- Pain

- Do not break blisters.
- Do not place ice directly on a burn.
- Do not chill the victim.

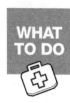

- Get medical attention immediately if the burned area is greater than one percent of the body, located over a joint, groin or on the face. If a small area is involved, immerse in fresh, cold water (preferably sterile water) or apply cold (ice/water) compresses over a clean cloth. Continue until pain subsides.
- Dry with a clean cloth and loosely cover with sterile non-stick dressing, protecting intact blisters. (Clean, clear food wrap or a plastic bag can also be used.)
- Elevate burned area.
- Get medical help.

Third-Degree Burns

SIGNS & SYMPTOMS:
- Damage to all layers of skin, including nerves
- Painless (because nerves have been damaged)
- White or black dry, leathery skin
- Possible charring of skin edges
- Area often surrounded by first- and second- degree burns

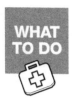

- Call for medical help.
- Monitor for responsiveness and breathing.
- Cover burn lightly with sterile non-stick dressing.
- Elevate burned area higher than victim's heart, if possible.
- If face is burned, have person sit up.
- Keep person warm and comfortable.
- Monitor and treat for *Shock*, if present.

HEAT BURNS

- Do not peel adhered clothing from burn.
- Do not rupture blisters.
- Do not apply ointment or household products to a burn, unless instructed by medical personnel.
- Do not apply ice directly to burn.
- Do not chill victim as you're cooling the burn area.

- Stop the burning process by removing ignited clothing and all jewelry from the burn area. Some items, such as belts, will continue to burn until removed.
- If extremities are burned, remove all jewelry beyond the burn, as swelling may develop and could cause the jewelry to cut off the circulation.
- Cool as soon as possible with drinkable water for at least 10 minutes.
- Give first aid for the degree of the burn.

CHEMICAL BURNS

Before an accident occurs, learn specific first aid procedures for any hazardous materials that you may possibly be exposed to. Check the emergency instructions on the container or consult the Material Safety Data Sheets (MSDS) or the **Poison Help Center** in your area.

SIGNS & SYMPTOMS:
- Red, irritated skin and eyes
- Burning sensation at contact area

- Do not try to neutralize chemical burns unless directed by professionals.
- Do not put any medicines or household products on a burn unless instructed by medical personnel.

- Be sure it is safe for you to help.
- Take steps to protect yourself from exposure to the chemical:
    - o Remove any contaminated clothing.
    - o In case of exposure to an acid or alkali on the skin, quickly pour copious amounts of water on area.
- Quickly flush chemical burns with lukewarm water (for at

least 10 minutes and then until pain subsides).
- Be sure to wash the chemical away completely.
- Treat *Chemical Burns of the Eye*(s) with immediate flushing with lukewarm water (for at least 15 minutes or until help arrives).
- All chemical burns - no matter how minor - require medical attention.

ELECTRICAL BURNS / SHOCK

Injury from exposure to electrical current can range from just a tingling sensation to *Shock* and death. You can't always tell from the outside what happened on the inside. Electricity passes through the body from entrance to exit wound, causing damage to any body part in its path - even causing the heart to beat irregularly or stop. For example, if a strong current has entered the hand and exited through the foot, the current has probably travelled through vital organs, causing serious injury. Electricity can cause: paralysis of the nerve centers, cessation of breathing, severe muscle spasm and breakage of bones.

If you come across an unconscious person lying near an electrical source, assume that the person is a victim of electric shock. All victims of electric shock and lightning strike need medical attention because not all injuries may be obvious.

SIGNS & SYMPTOMS:
- Loss of consciousness (sudden)
- Weak pulse
- Difficulty or no breathing
- Burns on the body (Two burn-like wounds may be evident - one where the current entered the body and one where it left)

- Do not touch a victim of electric shock who is still in contact with the source of power, or touch the wire itself - even an insulated part of the wire.
- Do not touch the victim until all wires are clear. A live, arcing wire may move, hitting you or someone else.
- Do not try to remove a high-voltage wire from the vicinity of the victim under any circumstances.

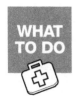

- Call EMS, the building's maintenance department or the utility company if a high-voltage wire is involved. Never attempt to remove it yourself.
- Make sure bystanders are aware of the existing danger.
- Cut the power at the source, if possible. At home, the switch is usually near the fuse box.
- If you can't turn power off at the source (and it's not a

high-voltage utility wire in contact with the victim), stand on a dry surface and disconnect victim from source of shock, using a long, non-conductive object, such as a fiberglass pole, broom, or rope.
- After source of shock has been removed, check the victim's responsiveness and breathing. Electricity can stop the heart! Perform CPR if needed.
- Monitor and treat for *Shock*, if present.
- Lightning can cause severe *Burns*, *Fractures* and even *Spinal Injury*, so treat for these injuries.
- If wounds are evident, cover wounds with dry sterile dressing.

CHEST PAIN

Discomfort described as 'pain' in the chest area can have many causes. Always think of a possible *Heart Attack* first. Lung infections (pneumonia), bronchitis, asthma, blood clots or a collapsed lung can all cause pain in the chest area. Trauma to the chest can fracture ribs and/or cause damage to underlying organs. Care at a recognized *Chest Pain Center* hospital can make a difference.

SIGNS & SYMPTOMS:
- Pain in the chest, which may be associated only with movement or breathing
- Fever, sweating, and paleness
- Cough
- Inability to breathe normally
- Anxiety

- Do not wait for pain to go away if victim's condition is worsening.
- Do not use age or personality to dismiss possible serious causes for the pain.
- Do not give victim anything to drink or eat.
- Do not give victim another person's medication unless told to do so by medical personnel.
- Do not leave the victim alone.

- Help victim find a comfortable position.
- Monitor the responsiveness and breathing.
- Get medical attention.

HEART ATTACK

Your heart muscle requires a steady supply of blood and oxygen. A heart attack occurs when that supply is interrupted or blocked. The release of a blood clot from hardened coronary arteries is often the culprit. Many illnesses, as well as drugs, especially cocaine and contraceptive pill usage, can cause a heart attack. Prompt medical attention can save heart muscles from dying. A blocked artery must be opened quickly by medications or surgery at a recognized *Chest Pain Center* hospital. Specialized care may include inducing hypothermia.

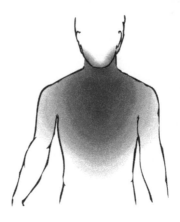

SIGNS & SYMPTOMS:
- Uncomfortable pressure, fullness or squeezing sensation in mid-chest, shoulder, jaw, back, stomach or arms
- Irregular heart rate (palpitations)
- Nausea, vomiting
- Sweating
- Pale, ashen skin
- Shortness of breath
- Anxiety, sense of impending doom

NOTE: Not all the signs and symptoms occur in every heart attack. Women, diabetics and the elderly often report vague and non-typical complaints.

- Do not attempt to relieve pain by walking or stretching.
- Do not force victim into uncomfortable position.
- Do not give anything by mouth except victim's prescription medication, such as nitroglycerin or aspirin.
- Do not leave victim alone.

WHAT TO DO

- Call for medical help. Time lost is muscle lost.

- If victim is unresponsive and not breathing:
    o Use *AED*, if immediately available.
    o If *AED* is unavailable, call for medical help before starting *CPR*.

- If responsive:
    o Loosen clothing and assist with victim's medication.
    o Comfort and reassure victim while keeping warm.
    o If you suspect it is heart pain and not contraindicated (e.g.: stroke, recent bleeding, or allergy), encourage the victim to chew 2 'baby' aspirins (low dose) or 1 adult aspirin. If uncertain, no aspirin.

- Monitor responsiveness and breathing until help arrives.

CHOKING

Choking is a life-threatening emergency. Every second counts. Often the victim will grab the throat with one or both hands when choking. Unless a victim is helped, loss of consciousness and death may follow. The action to clear a blocked airway is an abdominal thrust, also called the Heimlich maneuver practiced in first aid programs. Described below is the technique for a <u>conscious</u> choking victim who is **one year of age or older**. Different steps must be taken if the victim is unconscious or pregnant, or if the victim is less than one year of age. You can also learn the steps for these special situations in a first aid course.

SIGNS & SYMPTOMS:
- Inability to speak, cough or breathe
- Very weak cough, practically no sound made
- Grasping the throat - the universal choking sign of distress
- Noisy or high-pitched sounds
- Bluish lips or skin

DO NOT

- Do not use this procedure if the person is able to speak or cough.
- Do not leave a person who is trying to clear their throat or is weakly coughing alone.

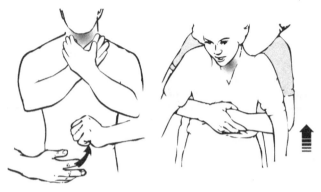

- Send someone to call for medical help.
- Ask "Are you choking?" If the victim only nods and can't speak, say "Can I help you?", say you are going to help.
- Kneel or stand behind the victim, bend the victim forward, and put both arms around waist.
- Make a fist with one hand, covering it with the other.
- Place thumb side of the fist against the abdomen, below the victim's breastbone, just above the navel.
- Grab the fist with your other hand, make an upward thrust into the abdomen, forcing the obstacle out.
- Repeat thrusts until the object has been dislodged or victim can breathe/cough.
- Get medical attention after the item has been dislodged, even if the victim says they are okay.
- If the victim becomes unconscious, start ***CPR***.

COLD EXPOSURE

Our bodies are affected by extremes in temperature. Shivering protects the chilled body by producing heat, but stops when we are very cold. Water in our skin and tissues can crystallize and freeze, causing abnormal function and sensation. Toes, nose, fingers and ears are especially sensitive to cold. Frostbite and hypothermia are the two emergencies associated with cold exposure.

Hypothermia can be life-threatening and must be treated immediately. It can take days for a rewarmed person to show signs of functioning.

FROSTBITE

SIGNS & SYMPTOMS:
- Cold, numb or painful skin
- Skin color progresses from white to yellow to gray
- Skin hard to the touch
- Skin does not move when you push on it

- Do not rub or massage the affected area.
- Do not break blisters.
- Do not give victim stimulants, including alcohol and tobacco.
- Do not leave victim alone. Frostbite can lead to hypothermia, which can lead to death.
- Do not place the affected body area in hot water.
- Do not use chemical warmers directly on frostbitten areas.
- Do not use stove, heating pad or fire to warm affected area.
- Do not thaw frozen part if a chance of refreezing exists or if near medical help.

- Move the victim to a warm area, cover with space blanket.
- Put affected body parts in warm water (100° - 105° F/ 37° - 40.6° C) until skin becomes flushed.
- After warming, keep affected fingers and toes separated with dry gauze.
- Give warm fluids.
- If normal sensations haven't returned within 30 minutes, get medical attention.

HYPOTHERMIA

SIGNS & SYMPTOMS:
Mild hypothermia
- Shivering
- Loss of coordination
- Confusion, irrational behavior
- Urge to urinate

Severe hypothermia

- No longer shivering, muscles stiff and rigid
- Stumbling
- Slow breathing
- Low blood pressure, weak pulse
- Slow, irregular heartbeat

- Do not leave victim alone.
- Do not use hot water to warm victim.
- Do not give hot liquids, alcohol, or anything by mouth.
- Do not move the victim unless necessary.
- Do not rub or massage the victim.

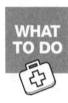

- Get victim out of the cold. Your goal is to prevent further heat loss and add warmth.
- Call for medical help. If victim is unresponsive and not breathing, an untrained rescuer should start **Chest Compressions** before rewarming.
- If you are far from medical care, start rewarming the victim. Rapid warming is required.
    o Remove any wet clothes, pat victim dry.
    o Cover victim's head, not face.
    o If possible, submerge victim's body in warm water (100° - 105° F/37°- 40° C) up to the chin.
    o If unable to submerge victim, use a space blanket or your own body heat to warm victim.
    o Apply warm - not hot - packs to neck, armpits and groin. Reapply as packs become cool.
- Stay with the victim, warming them while monitoring responsiveness and breathing until help arrives.
- If victim must be moved, do so gently, keeping the victim in a horizontal position.

DENTAL / MOUTH INJURY

Injuries to the mouth area, including jaw and teeth, can have a good outcome if simple first aid techniques are used. Bleeding from the mouth can be serious if the airway and breathing is blocked by blood or knocked-out teeth. Lips can bleed and swell quickly due to a rich blood supply.

SIGNS & SYMPTOMS:
- Pain, swelling
- Bleeding
- Inability to close mouth

• Trouble breathing

•   Do not force the jaw open or closed.
•   Do not pull a tooth that is partially out.
•   Do not handle the part of the tooth that was in the gum.
•   Do not use force to reinsert tooth.
•   Do not try to stop bleeding if you can't see the source.

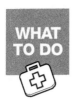

If difficulty speaking or breathing:
•   Call for medical help
•   Place victim in a position of comfort

If bleeding from the mouth and no loose or missing teeth are visible:
•   Put gloves on and apply pressure to visible bleeding area with gauze or clean cloth. Apply cold pack (mixture ice/water) to swelling.
•   If bleeding is deep in the mouth, place victim in *Recovery Position* to prevent victim from choking on blood.
•   Get medical help if bleeding can't be stopped or victim has trouble breathing.
•   Monitor and treat for *Shock*, if present.

If tooth is loose:
•   Have victim gently bite down on sterile gauze to keep tooth in place
•   Get dental help.

If a tooth is knocked out:
•   Handle the tooth by the crown.
•   If tooth can go in easily, gently reinsert into socket.
•   If not, rinse tooth in water and place in solution that preserves, such as Hank's balanced salt solution, propolis, whole milk, coconut water, or egg white. This will extend the viability of the tooth.
•   Take victim and tooth to dentist as quickly as possible.
•   Clean any bleeding wounds with tap water.
•   **Stop bleeding from gum** by applying pressure with a piece of cotton or gauze for at least five minutes, using increased pressure if needed.

EAR INJURY

Injury and/or pain in the ear, no matter what the cause, require medical attention. An ear problem may be from the inner, middle or outer ear. The eardrum can rupture from a direct blow, infection, loud noise or deep dive. Dirt and bacteria from the outer canal can travel into the inner ear, causing an infection. Drainage from the ear can also be a sign of a head injury. Ear conditions can affect hearing and balance and cause dizziness.

SIGNS & SYMPTOMS:
- Pain, earache
- Headache
- Jaw pain or tooth pain
- Swelling, drainage
- Hearing problems
- Nausea, vomiting
- Dizziness, vertigo, loss of balance

- Do not attempt to remove any object from the ear canal unless you can see it clearly.
- Do not block any drainage coming from the ear.
- Do not attempt to clean drainage within the ear canal.
- Do not move the victim if you suspect neck or spinal injury.
- Do not assume an amputated ear piece cannot be reattached.
- Do not let a victim put anything in the ear, including a finger, to get something out.

INJURY TO THE OUTER EAR

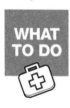

- If you suspect *Head Trauma*, call for medical help.
- If *Bleeding*, apply direct pressure.
- If a portion has been amputated, follow steps for treating *Amputation*.
- Apply cool compress to decrease swelling.
- Get medical attention.

FOREIGN BODY IN EAR

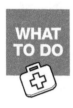

- Stay calm and reassure the victim.
- Look inside ear with a flashlight.
- If you can see the foreign body:
  - If victim is cooperative, use tweezers to remove the item.
  - If unsuccessful, tilt head with affected ear facing down.

- If you can't see the foreign body:
  - Do not try to remove it.
  - Tilt head with affected ear facing down.
- If you suspect the object is an insect:
  - Avoid head movement.
  - An insect will crawl up, so tilt the affected ear up instead.
- Get medical attention.

RUPTURED EARDRUM / EAR DRAINAGE

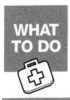

WHAT TO DO

- If you suspect *Head Trauma* as the cause, get medical help.
- Cover outside ear with loose, dry sterile dressing.
- Have the victim lie on side with affected ear facing down if there's no sign of head or neck injury.
- Get medical attention.

EYE INJURY

Injuries to the eye - no matter what the cause - require immediate medical attention. When irritated by any substance, however, the eye should be washed for at least 20 minutes before going for medical attention or while waiting for medical assistance to arrive. Eye injuries can be frightening for the victim. Be sure to calm and assure the victim as best you can. Eye pain can also be caused by medical problems, such as glaucoma, so always get medical attention for eye pain.

SIGNS & SYMPTOMS:
- Pain
- Excess blinking, tearing
- Bleeding, redness, swelling
- Vision problems
- Sensitivity to light

DO NOT

- Do not attempt to remove an object from the eye with any liquid other than sterile eyewash or clean water.
- Do not delay in washing an irritant from the eye.
- Do not attempt to pull out any object stuck in the eyeball.
- Do not rub painful eye(s).
- Never apply pressure to the eyeball, even to stop bleeding.

OBJECT IN EYE

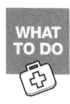

- Flush eye:
  - Use sterile eyewash or clean water.
  - Gently flush from the inner area of the eye next to the nose to the outer area.
  - As you flush, pull down lower lid and lift the upper lid.
  - Ask victim to roll eyes around.
- Get medical attention if the object isn't removed or irritation persists.

CHEMICAL BURNS OF THE EYE

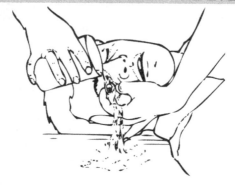

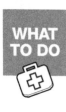

- Don't delay. Begin flushing immediately. Hold the lids open and pour fresh water over eye or position under slowly running water. Water should flow from the inner area of the eye next to the nose to the outer area, to avoid contamination of the other eye.
- Flush with copious amounts of tap water for at least 15 continuous minutes or until medical help arrives.
- Contact **Poison Help Center**. Get medical attention for any chemical burns of the eyes.

CUTS OF THE EYE OR EYELID

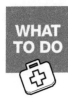

- Gently apply dry sterile bandage and clean cold compress to area.
- Keep both eyes closed.
- Get medical attention immediately.

OBJECT IMPALED IN EYE

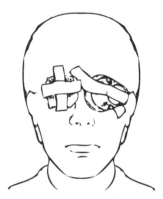

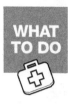

WHAT TO DO

- Cover object protruding from eyeball without touching either the eye or the object, using a paper cup or similar object that won't disturb the imbedded object.
- Cover both eyes with dry sterile dressing to prevent natural movement by injured eye.
- Get medical attention immediately.

GENITAL INJURY

Pain in the genital area can be caused by trauma or internal disease. Bleeding in this area can be serious and can cause **Shock** and even death. If a foreign body is suspected, do not try to remove it. Seek medical attention. Proper tools and knowledge of anatomy will ensure no further damage is done.

SIGNS & SYMPTOMS:
- Pain
- *Bleeding*
- Pale skin
- Bruising, swelling
- *Shock*

DO NOT

- Do not force victim into uncomfortable position.
- Do not give anything by mouth in case surgery is needed.
- Do not try to remove any stuck objects.

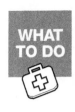

- Call for medical help if unable to control **Bleeding** or victim is unable to move.
- Find position of comfort.
- If pale and bleeding, place victim in **Shock Position** until help arrives.
- Apply cold pack (mixture ice/water) to area if there is swelling and bleeding has stopped.
- Get medical attention.

HEAD TRAUMA

The brain is cushioned by spinal fluid and encased in the skull. Direct trauma to the head may cause many types of injuries, including a fractured skull, bleeding of the scalp or a bruise of the brain. Head trauma, although usually minor, can be a serious emergency. If any head injury causes change in alertness, progressive signs of concussion or other causes for concern, seek medical help.

SIGNS & SYMPTOMS:
- Headache, dizziness
- Bleeding or bump on head
- Nausea, vomiting
- Fluid seeping from ear and nose
- Sleepiness
- Inappropriate behavior
- **Unconsciousness** or unresponsiveness for seconds to hours
- Unequal pupils (black spot in eye)
- **Seizures**

- Do not move a victim's head if a spinal injury is suspected.
- Do not give anything by mouth.
- Do not try to keep victim awake.

- Call for medical help.
- If absolutely necessary to turn victim, turn as unit. Use two rescuers and the **Log-Roll Technique.**
- If absolutely necessary to move victim, use **Clothes-Drag Technique**.
- Immobilize neck and head if spine or neck injury is suspected.
- Monitor for responsiveness and breathing.
- Control **Bleeding**, if present.
- Watch for signs of serious head trauma, such as

increasing sleepiness, projectile vomiting, *Seizures* and loss of body function control.
- Keep victim calm and still until help arrives.

HEAT EXPOSURE

The body functions best within a narrow temperature range. High temperatures increase the body's metabolic rate and decrease its efficiency. Loss of fluid and dilation of blood vessels occur in an attempt to cool down. Being elderly and/or taking certain medications can place you at increased risk for heat illness. The two major medical emergencies associated with heat exposure are heat exhaustion and heatstroke.

HEAT EXHAUSTION

SIGNS & SYMPTOMS:
- Sweating, moist, clammy skin
- Muscle cramps, weakness and fatigue
- Nausea, vomiting
- Slightly elevated body temperature
- Headache
- Dizziness

- Do not ignore symptoms. If untreated, heat-related illnesses get worse.
- Do not give victim any stimulant, including alcohol or cigarettes.
- Do not apply ice directly to skin.
- Do not allow victim to become so cold that they shiver when cooling.
- Do not leave victim alone.
- Do not use rubbing alcohol or anything other than water on the victim's skin.

- Remove victim from heat.
- Sponge or spray with cool water. Fan victim. Stop if victim develops goose bumps or shivers.
- If victim is conscious and can take fluids, have victim drink 16 oz./0.5 L of electrolyte/carbohydrate mixture, juice or milk every 30 minutes until recovered.
- Get medical attention if person doesn't continually improve.

HEATSTROKE

SIGNS & SYMPTOMS:
- Hot, dry skin
- Red or spotted skin
- Inability to drink
- Shallow breathing
- Extremely high body temperature
- Mental confusion, strange behavior
- ***Seizures***
- Loss of consciousness

- Do not ignore symptoms. If untreated, heat-related illnesses get worse.
- Do not wait to start cooling the victim.
- Do not force fluids.
- Do not give victim aspirin or any other medication to lower temperature.
- Do not give victim any stimulant, including alcohol or cigarettes.
- Do not apply ice directly to skin.
- Do not allow victim to become so cold that they shiver.
- Do not leave victim alone.

- Call for medical help.
- Remove person from heat whenever possible.
- Remove victim's clothing and place them in a cool bath up to the chin (if possible), or apply cool compresses to neck, armpits and groin.
- If victim becomes unresponsive and stops breathing, start ***CPR***.
- Medical attention is always required.

NOSE BLEED

A nose bleed is often caused by a direct blow to the face or head, high blood pressure problems or the use of blood thinning medications, including aspirin. It's hard to know how much bleeding occurs during a nose bleed because the victim often swallows some blood.

SIGNS & SYMPTOMS:
- Bleeding from one or both nostrils
- Spitting up or vomiting blood
- Headache, fullness of the sinuses and ears
- Trouble breathing

- Do not ask the victim to lean their head back.
- Do not use an ice pack on the nose or forehead.
- Do not press on the bone/bridge of the nose between the eyes.
- Do not pinch nostrils and press into face if broken face bones are suspected.

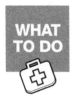

WHAT TO DO

- Put on gloves or find a barrier for your hands.
- Have victim sit, leaning forward, and gently blow out blood clots. Immediately pinch together the soft part of both nostrils while pushing into the face bone.
- Continue constant pressure for 5 minutes, pinching harder if bleeding persists.
- Seek medical assistance if you're unable to control the bleeding after 15 minutes, or if bleeding is heavy or the victim has trouble breathing.

POISONING EMERGENCY

Poisoning may be accidental or intentional - drugs, chemicals and household cleaners are all potential poisons. They can hurt or kill you! Children are the most common victims of accidental poisoning. Adults and adolescents sometimes use poison to end their lives. A poison or toxin can affect the individual through skin contact, injection, *Fume Inhalation* or swallowing. Know the number of your local **Poison Help Center**. Remember, in the United States call 1-800-222-1222. All questions about poisons are smart questions.

SIGNS & SYMPTOMS:
- Nausea, vomiting
- Headache
- Altered consciousness
- Abdominal pain
- Local irritation at site of exposure (eye, skin, airway)

- Do not rely solely on a container's label for first aid information.
- Do not force vomiting or give fluids to victim unless told to by a physician or the **Poison Help Center**. Be sure the victim is totally conscious beforehand.
- Do not assume everyone wants to get well. Don't leave a victim alone if attempted suicide is suspected.

- Call for medical help.
- Protect yourself from exposure to the poison while administering first aid.
- For poison in the eye, follow instructions for ***Chemical Burns of the Eyes.***
- For poison on the skin, take off any clothing that the poison touched and rinse the skin with running water for at least 20 minutes, continuing until any irritation subsides.
- For inhaled poison, move the victim to fresh air right away. Monitor for ***Breathing Problems.***
- Call **Poison Help Center** for specific instructions. They will want to know:
  o Type of poison
  o How it happened
  o Age of victim
  o Estimated amount and time at which poisoning occurred
  o Victim's condition
- Follow **Poison Help Center's** instructions!

SEIZURES

A seizure is often described as haphazard electrical discharges of the brain that cause parts of the body to move erratically. There are a number of things that can trigger a seizure. Seizures are often the result of illness, head injury, stroke, aneurysm, low blood sugar, poisoning or high fever. Children up to age 5 are especially prone to fever-related seizures. Your role as rescuer is to make sure the victim doesn't get hurt. Seizure activity can appear in many different ways. Seizures will almost always spontaneously stop, and the victim will have a period of drowsiness, confusion or sleep before gradual awakening.

SIGNS & SYMPTOMS:
- Unresponsiveness
- Loss of muscle control with jerking motion of one or many parts of the body
- Loss of control of body functions
- Duration seconds to minutes

- Do not force any object between victim's teeth.
- Do not hold victim down.
- Do not throw water on victim in an attempt to stop seizure or awaken.
- Do not leave victim alone.

- Call for medical help.
- Prevent injury by removing objects that the victim could strike. Place cushioning material around victim, if possible.
- Stay with victim, monitoring for *Breathing Problems*.
- If victim bites his tongue and is bleeding, wait for seizure to stop before giving first aid for *Bleeding*.
- If you do not suspect head, neck or spine injury, place victim in *Recovery Position* after seizure has stopped.
- If fever is the cause, treat by cooling until alert enough to take medication to lower temperature.
- Monitor for responsiveness and breathing.
- Seek medical attention.

SHOCK

Any serious injury or illness can result in shock, which is a life-threatening condition. Shock can develop quickly or gradually. It is a failure of the heart and blood vessels to provide enough oxygen to every part of the body. Without oxygen, the various body systems - especially the heart, brain and the kidneys - will begin to slow down and ultimately die. The degree of shock is determined by a number of factors, including:

- Age (especially high in the very young and very old)
- Victim's general health
- Excessive fatigue
- Rough handling
- Delay of medical attention

SIGNS & SYMPTOMS:

- Anxiety, restlessness
- Rapid, weak pulse
- Rapid, shallow breathing
- Pale, cold, clammy skin
- Blue/pale lips and nail beds
- Coldness of extremities
- Thirst, dryness in mouth
- Nausea
- Dizziness, fainting
- Mental confusion

DO NOT

- Do not elevate victim's head if spine or leg injury is suspected.
- Do not give victim anything to eat or drink.

- Call for medical help.
- Control **Bleeding.**
- Check and monitor responsiveness and breathing.
- Place in **Shock Position.**
- Keep victim warm until help arrives.

SPINAL INJURY

A spinal injury isn't always obvious. Suspect one with injuries to the face or neck. Spinal injuries are often the result of falls, diving, electrocution or motor vehicle or sports accidents. Always suspect a spinal injury until determined otherwise, especially if a person is not totally alert or under the influence of alcohol or drugs.

SIGNS & SYMPTOMS:
- Back or neck pain
- Tingling or weakness in arms or legs
- Any trauma to head, back or chest
- Loss of sensation and function of extremities
- Change in level of responsiveness or alertness after an injury

- Do not turn or move victim unless there's a danger of fire, explosion or other life-threatening incident.
- Do not put pillow under victim's head.
- Do not give victim anything to eat or drink.

- Call for medical help.
- ONLY if victim needs to be turned on back, use **Log-Roll Technique.**
- ONLY if victim is in imminent danger, use **Clothes-Drag Technique** to move victim to safety. Hold the head and neck so that they do not move, bend or twist.
- Immobilize the head and neck in the position found. Use your hands, blankets, clothing or any other available materials to hold head and neck firmly.
- Calm and reassure victim until help arrives.

STROKE

A stroke occurs when a blood vessel to the brain or within the brain bursts or becomes blocked and no blood can flow to brain tissue. When blood flow stops, brain tissue begins to die. Time lost is brain lost! Clot-busting drugs, if given within 3 - 4.5 hours, or clot removal within 6 - 16 hours and up to 24 hours, can open some blocked arteries. Remember: hours includes the time for medical evaluation. Every minute counts, so immediate medical attention is important. Your role as a rescuer is to recognize the signs and symptoms of a stroke and help get the victim to *a Stroke Center* hospital fast.

A Transient Ischemic Attack (TIA), also called "warning stroke" or "mini-stroke", causes signs and symptoms just like a stroke, but they go away. This is a sign that a full-blown stroke may be on the way. TIAs should not be ignored, even if symptoms go away quickly.

SIGNS & SYMPTOMS:
- Sudden unexplained dizziness/trouble walking
- Sudden intense headache, "worst headache ever"
- Sudden dimness or loss of vision, usually in one eye
- Sudden inability to speak, slurred or incoherent speech
- Sudden loss of sensation and/or function on one side of the face, arms or legs
- Sudden confusion, *Unconsciousness*

Perform a FAST Test:
Face: Ask the person to smile. If one side droops, it may be a TIA or stroke.

Arms: Ask the person to hold out both arms in front of the body. If one arm droops, it may be a TIA or stroke.

Speech: Ask the person to repeat a simple sentence. If speech is slurred or garbled, or other errors occur, it may be a stroke or TIA.

Time: If any of these happens, call for medical help. Ask for the nearest *Stroke Center* hospital.

- Do not give victim anything to eat or drink.
- Do not delay getting medical attention.

- Call for medical help immediately.
- Monitor responsiveness and breathing.
- Calm and reassure victim until help arrives.
- Have victim rest in a comfortable position.
- If the victim loses consciousness, place in the *Recovery Position*.
- Stay with the victim until help arrives.

UNCONSCIOUSNESS

This is an abnormal state of awareness in which the victim cannot be aroused. There are different levels, ranging from drowsiness to coma. The victim need not be motionless. Loss of consciousness can be brief, as in fainting. Low blood sugar, head trauma and poisoning are just a few of the conditions that can result in unconsciousness. Always be sure the person isn't sleeping before calling for medical assistance.

SIGNS & SYMPTOMS:
- Drowsy, sleepy, disoriented or incoherent
- Motionless and silent
- Does not respond to strong touch and loud voice

- Do not give victim anything to eat or drink.
- Do not move if any sign of trauma - cuts, bumps or bleeding.
- Do not leave victim alone.
- Do not try to wake with water on face or slapping.
- Do not put pillow under head; this position could block the airway.

- Call for medical help.
- Look for causes of unconsciousness.
- Monitor responsiveness and breathing.
- Monitor for *Seizures.*
- If there is no possibility that the victim has a head or spinal injury, place in *Recovery Position*.
- If low blood sugar is suspected:
  - Check blood sugar level, if possible.
  - If victim can follow commands and swallow safely, give glucose tablets (preferable), orange juice, soft chewy candy or fruit leather - not sugar substitutes).
  - Assist victim with their injection of glucagon for treating low blood sugar.
  - Re-check sugar level 15-20 minutes after treatment.
- Stay with the victim until help arrives.

5. EMERGENCY FIRST AID TECHNIQUES

In this section, you'll find out some of the emergency first aid techniques suggested in this guide. Again, keep in mind that there's a difference between reading about the techniques and practicing them under the guidance of a first aid instructor. Reading about first aid is no substitute for first aid training.

Positioning a victim should only be done to avoid danger or to provide care.

Only change position if victim is:
- *Unconscious*
- In immediate danger in current location
- Breathing and unresponsive
- Vomiting or has debris in mouth
- In *Shock*

Remember - Do No Further Harm!

LOG-ROLL TECHNIQUE

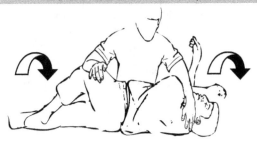

This technique allows you to safely turn a victim who is lying face down, if they are having difficulty breathing and there is no suspicion of spinal trauma.
Remember, it is important to roll the person as a unit.
If you have assistance, stabilize the head and neck while you instruct your helper to roll the victim's body as a single unit onto their back or into the *Recovery Position*.

If you are alone:
- Kneel at the waistline area of the victim.
- Attempt to roll the victim as a single unit by grasping the opposite shoulder and opposite hip and rolling the victim towards you.
- As soon as movement begins, take your hand from the shoulder to support the head and neck area until the victim is in the lateral side-lying position or the *Recovery Position*.

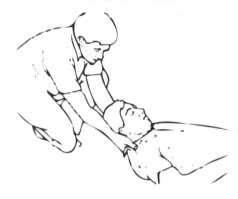

If you're alone and a victim absolutely has to be moved, follow these steps:

- Lay victim on back and put your hands under the victim's shoulders, grabbing victim's clothing. Be careful not to cause an airway obstruction by pulling the clothing too tightly.
- Support victim's head, keeping the head as close to the floor as possible.
- Drag the victim by their clothing, keeping the body aligned. Pull as a unit; hold the head and neck as one, so no bending or twisting occurs.

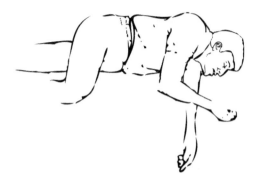

If spinal injury is suspected, DO NOT move or put victim in recovery position. A victim who is unresponsive but breathing normally should be placed in lateral lying position. Bend both legs to stabilize. Side-lying positions help prevent any blood or vomit from getting into the victim's lungs. Victims left alone should be in this position.

SHOCK POSITION

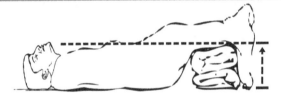

Do not put victim in this position if spinal injury is suspected. Place a responsive victim, breathing normally, with signs of shock in this position. Only do so if there is no evidence of trauma or injury and it does not cause pain. This may help to increase return blood flow to the heart.

- Lay victim on back. Don't place pillow under head.
- Elevate legs (if not painful) above a minimum of 6 to12 in/15-30 cm (about 30°-60°) above head level.
- Cover to maintain body temperature and keep victim comfortable.

6. EMERGENCY INFO SHEET (EIS)

Take the time now to fill in all the necessary information the EMS dispatcher will need to know so that you'll be ready to act quickly and correctly in the event of an emergency.

1. FIRST AID KIT

Nearest AED_____

2. EMERGENCY TELEPHONE NUMBERS
(Put a star next to the phone number that should be called first in your area.)

EMERGENCY MEDICAL SERVICES - EMS (911 in the USA/Canada)

PERSONAL DOCTOR

FIRE DEPARTMENT

POLICE

POISON HELP CENTER (1-800-222-1222 in USA)

NEAREST HOSPITAL

Directions:

3. WHEN YOU CALL FOR HELP, BE READY TO PROVIDE THE FOLLOWING INFORMATION

YOUR NAME

TYPE OF EMERGENCY

    Number Injured _____

LOCATION OF EMERGENCY

Street address/apartment number

Cross streets/nearby landmarks

Major intersections

Telephone number you're calling from

4. DESCRIBE WHAT HAPPENED
You can be given instructions on how to help until EMS arrives. Someone should be available to relay instructions if the emergency is not near a telephone.

5. STAY ON THE PHONE UNTIL TOLD IT IS OKAY TO HANG UP

7. FIRST AID KIT CHECKLIST

- Keep a first aid kit in the home, workplace and car.
- Let everyone concerned know where it is.
- Carry the first aid kit when you go to help anyone.
- Restock after using.

CHECKLIST
- *Doc's First Aid Guide* with completed ***Emergency Info Sheet***

Equipment
- CPR barrier mask (face shield)
- Cotton swabs
- Cold pack
- Paper cups
- Space blanket
- Thermometer
- Plastic bags able to be sealed

Medication
- Antiseptic wipes/towelettes
- Sterile eye wash with eye cup
- Antiseptic/anesthetic spray
- Antibiotic ointment
- Calamine/antihistamine lotion
- Activated Charcoal tablets/powder

Instruments
- Tweezers
- Blunt tipped scissors
- Bulb syringe

Miscellaneous
- Disposable gloves
- Change for a pay phone
- Candles, waterproof matches
- Pocket flashlight
- Paper/pencil
- Packet tissues
- Soap
- Safety pin

Dressings
- Sterile cotton balls
- Sterile eye patches
- Sterile gauze pads
- Hypoallergenic adhesive tape
- Elastic bandage
- Roller bandage
- Sterile non-stick pads
- Absorbent compress
- Adhesive bandage strips
- Triangular bandages
- Butterfly bandages